Yosra Yahia
Abdelwahab Mghirbi
Jihène Guissouma

Acute respiratory failure in the elderly in the emergency room

Yosra Yahia
Abdelwahab Mghirbi
Jihène Guissouma

Acute respiratory failure in the elderly in the emergency room

Difficulties of non-invasive ventilatory treatment and predictive factors

ScienciaScripts

Imprint

Any brand names and product names mentioned in this book are subject to trademark, brand or patent protection and are trademarks or registered trademarks of their respective holders. The use of brand names, product names, common names, trade names, product descriptions etc. even without a particular marking in this work is in no way to be construed to mean that such names may be regarded as unrestricted in respect of trademark and brand protection legislation and could thus be used by anyone.

Cover image: www.ingimage.com

This book is a translation from the original published under ISBN 978-620-3-44095-9.

Publisher:
Sciencia Scripts
is a trademark of
Dodo Books Indian Ocean Ltd. and OmniScriptum S.R.L Publishing group
Str. Armeneasca 28/1, office 1, Chisinau MD-2012, Republic of Moldova, Europe
Printed at: see last page
ISBN: 978-620-5-24464-7

TABLE OF CONTENTS

INTRODUCTION

Emergency departments are receiving an increasing number of elderly patients (1). This can be explained in part by the significant aging of the population (2).

The World Health Organization (WHO) defines an "elderly person" as a person older than 65 years (2). However, the new definitions tend to evolve towards an estimation of physiological age, taking into account the presence or absence of co-morbidities, which would allow a better appreciation of the aging of the organism (2).

Because of the greater frequency of chronic respiratory and/or cardiovascular disease, elderly patients often present to the emergency department with acute respiratory failure (ARF). This is an extreme emergency in which the patient presents with clinical signs of acute respiratory distress, which may be accompanied by signs of cardiac failure and neuropsychological signs of impaired hematosis and tissue oxygenation.The therapeutic management of these patients takes place mainly in the emergency room and must be rapid and effective, because the vital prognosis is imminently committed. The therapeutic approach, as for patients of any age, is based on the initiation of an adapted ventilatory treatment, whose goal is to improve gas exchange while decreasing the work of breathing. This treatment must be associated with a medicinal treatment which depends on the etiology of the ARF.In the elderly, etiologies are often associated, which can complicate the therapeutic management of ARF. Among the ventilatory supports, non-invasive ventilation (NIV) can be an alternative, allowing to avoid as much as possible the complications of invasive ventilation. This ventilatory modality includes all mechanical respiratory assistance techniques that do not require an endotracheal approach by intubation or tracheostomy. It is commonly referred to as non-invasive positive pressure ventilation in which the patient and ventilator are connected by a mask or mouthpiece (3).

The efficacy of NIV has been widely established during acute heart failure (AHF) and acute decompensation of chronic obstructive pulmonary disease (CAD) (4).

In emergency departments, NIV is increasingly practiced, especially in the elderly, where it is in some cases the only alternative for respiratory assistance offered in the context of a limitation of therapeutic care.Although this technique is commonly used for the management of ARF in the elderly in the emergency department, specific data remain limited regarding its effectiveness in this population. The objectives of this work are to study the characteristics of non-invasive ventilatory therapy in the elderly subject admitted to the emergency department for ARF and to highlight the predictive factors.

METHODS

I- The method

I.1. Type of study

This is a retrospective study conducted in the emergency department of the university hospital La Rabta.

I.2. Description of the study site

The emergency department of the CHU La Rabta attracts patients from all over Tunis and even from other regions of the national territory, with a number of consultants of 100,000 per year. It includes several sectors arranged:

o A patient reception room opening at the entrance of the department.

o A triage unit where an emergency nurse organizer (ENO) performs the initial assessment of each patient by measuring vital signs and recording them on a patient observation form. An electrocardiogram (ECG) is performed depending on the clinical context. At the end of this evaluation, the IOA refers the patient according to the reason for consultation and the presence or absence of signs of gravity.

o A level B life-saving emergency room for patients with an acute pathology deemed reversible requiring care and monitoring for a few hours in the absence of vital distress requiring resuscitation.

o A trauma room

o A room for biological samples and the administration of treatments

o A standard radiology room

o One surgery consultation room and two medicine consultation rooms o And finally, a hospitalization service with two intensive care rooms for patients requiring intensive care and three observation rooms forming the UHCD or short-term hospitalization unit.

In practice, patients with signs of ARF are rapidly transferred to the department's resuscitation rooms.

I.3. The study period

This study was conducted over a period of one year and four months, from January 2017 to April 2018.

I.4. Patient selection criteria

- Inclusion criteria:

All patients older than sixty-five years admitted to the emergency department for AKI requiring NIV were included.

- Non-inclusion criteria: Not included in our study were:

Patients put on NIV for the purpose of pre-oxygenation or weaning from mechanical ventilation.

- Exclusion Criteria:

Patients with missing data were excluded

I.5. Data collection

The data were collected from the hospital records on a pre-established form including:

- Sociodemographic parameters: age, gender, history and Charlson index calculated for all patients to assess comorbidities (see appendix).

- Clinical parameters at admission: pleuropulmonary, cardiovascular, neurological and general examination (temperature)
- Paraclinical parameters provided by the initial blood gas (ABG), the rest of the biological workup, electrocardiogram (ECG), and chest radiograph.

Data were then entered and analyzed using SPSS version 22 software.

II- The practice of non-invasive ventilation

II.1. Modes and respirators

▪ Inspiratory support mode
During the study period, the Inspiratory Support mode was applied using Taema, Newport and Covidien ventilators.

This mode allows to deliver two levels of pressure in spontaneous ventilation (SV) during the two breathing times, namely an inspiratory aid (IA) and a positive expiratory pressure (PEP).

For the inspiratory trigger, a cutoff of 2L/min was usually set.

FiO2 is adjusted to the therapeutic target oxygenation goals. Similarly, the ventilatory parameters: AI, PEEP, slope and expiratory trigger are adapted to the causative pathology and the patient's clinical response.

This is assessed by continuous monitoring of expiratory tidal volume (ETV), expiratory minute volume (EMV) and respiratory rate, displayed on the ventilator. A target ETV of 6 to 8 ml/kg is recommended (5,6). Similarly, continuous scopic monitoring of peripheral oxygen saturation (SpO2), heart rate (HR), and electrocardiographic tracing is instituted during the NIV session with measurement of blood pressure every four hours and monitoring of other clinical parameters, in particular neurological status and arterial gasometry.

▪ The CPAP mode (or continuous positive airway pressure)

This mode, which provides continuous PEEP, is applied by means of a Boussignac valve with a manometer available to monitor the PEEP level.

II.2. The interface

In our department, it is done by means of a naso-buccal mask whose size is adapted to the morphology of the patient in order to prevent leaks. This mask is then fixed by means of a harness in such a way as to ensure its watertightness and to respect the patient's comfort after having explained the procedure to him, the expected benefit and having left him a time of adaptation.

III- Statistical analysis

It was descriptive in the first instance with the calculation of absolute and relative frequencies for the qualitative variables. We also calculated means and standard deviations for the quantitative variables.Comparisons of two means on independent series were performed using the Student's t-test for independent series and, in case of non-validity, by the non-parametric Mann-Whithney test.Comparisons of percentages on independent series were made by Pearson's chi-square test, and in case of invalidity of this test, by Fisher's exact test.NIV failure was defined by the use of orotracheal intubation, ICU hospitalization, and in-hospital mortality.The analytical study focused on the correlation between clinical and biological parameters at admission and in-hospital mortality. The threshold of significance was set at 0.05.Figures and diagrams illustrating the main results were produced using SPSS software.

IV-Bibliographic research

The engines of search engines were: PubMed, Science Direct and CochraneWe used the following keywords:

- The ventilation non invasive ventilation, subject elderly subject,emergencies, acute respiratory failure, dyspnea

- Non invasive ventilation, elderly, old patients, acute respiratory failure, emergency, positive airway pressure ventilation, Bilevel, CPAP.

RESULTS

During the study period, we collected 75 patients.

I- Characteristics of the study population

I.1. Demographic characteristics

Our population had a clear male predominance with 72% men (n=54), 28% women (n=21) and a sex ratio of 2.57.The median age of the population was 74 years with a minimum age of 65 years and a maximum age of 88 years. The very old subjects, i.e. those over 75 years of age, represented 50.7% of the population.

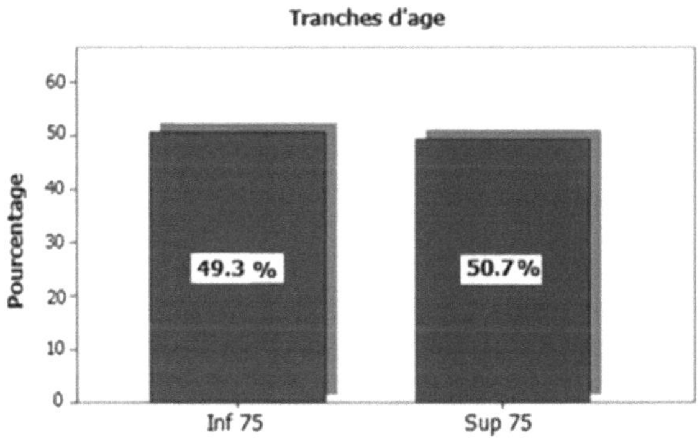

Figure 1: Distribution of the population by over and under 75 years

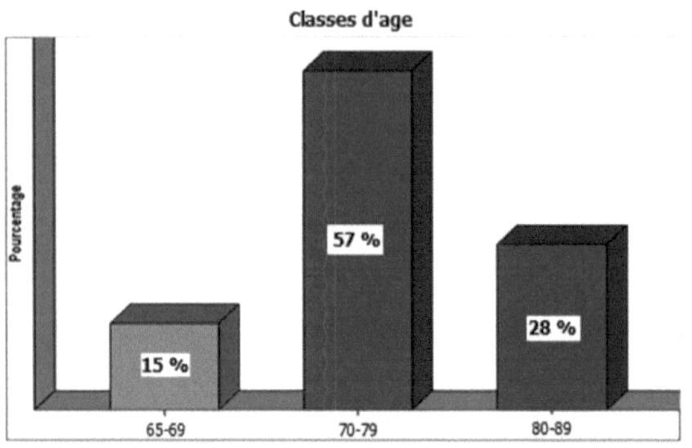

Figure 2: Distribution of the population by age group

The age category of 70-79 years included more than half of the patients or 57%.

I.2. Clinical characteristics

The clinical characteristics of the population a t admission are represented in the following tables (Tables I, II and III):

Table I: Patient history

Background	% (N=75)
HTA	51
COPD	67
Heart failure	29
ACFA	28
Coronary insufficiency	20
Renal insufficiency	27
Diabetes	35
STROKE	8

AH: high blood pressure; COPD: chronic obstructive pulmonary disease;
AFCA: atrial fibrillation cardiac arrhythmia; stroke: cerebrovascular accident

The Charlson index had a median value of 5. The minimum value was 3 and the maximum was 9.

Table II: Initial assessment of vital parameters

Vital signs	Workforce	%
SpO2 (%)		
90-94	7	9,3
86-89	24	32
80-85	16	21,3
<80	28	37,3
FR (c/mn)		
>30c/min	41	55
25-30 c/min	26	34
20-24	5	7
<20	3	4
SAP (mmHg)		
>180	11	15
<100	1	1,3
DBP (mmHg)		
≤40	0	0
>90	9	12
Heart rate (c/min)		
>120	20	27
90-120	46	61
<90	9	12
Temperature >38°C	15	20
SG		
15	53	71
9-14	17	22
≤8	5	7

SpO2: peripheral oxygen saturation; RF: respiratory rate; SBP: systolic blood pressure; DBP: diastolic blood pressure; GCS: Glasgow score

Table III: Other clinical signs

Clinical signs	%
Signs of struggle	83
Crackling rales	48
Sibling Rails	63,5
Snoring Rales	23
TSJ	32
IMO	45
RHJ	17

TSJ: spontaneous jugular turgidity; OMI: lower extremity edema; RHJ: hepato-jugular reflux

Data from the analysis of blood samples at admission (Biology and GDS) are summarized in the following tables (Tables IV and V):

Table IV: Biology data at admission

Biological blood tests	Workforce	%
Urea (g/L)		
≤0,45	21	28
>0,46	52	70
Creatinine (mg/L)		
≤12	36	48
>12	37	49
NFS		
Hemoglobin < 10 g/dL	9	10
WBC >10000/mm3	49	65
WBC <4000/mm3	5	7
CRP > 10mg/L	51	68

CBC: blood count; WBC: white blood cells; CRP: C-reactive protein

Table V: Admission Blood Gas Analysis

GDS	Average value
pH	7,32 (±0,08)
PaCO2 (mmHg)	61 (±22)
HCO3 (mmoles/L)	30,4 (±10,4)

GDS: blood gas; PaCO2: arterial carbon dioxide pressure; HCO3: blood bicarbonate level

Chest X-ray analysis showed unilateral alveolar-interstitial syndrome in 18%, bilateral in 48% and pleural effusion in 27%.The electrical abnormalities present at admission were repolarization disorders (65%), atrial fibrillation cardiac arrhythmia (21%), branch block-type conductive disorders (12%), and excitability disorders (5%).Acute respiratory failure was hypercapnic in 71% and non-hypercapnic in 39%.

II- Etiologies of acute respiratory failure

The etiological diagnoses of AKI were DABPCO in 72% of cases, CIA in 61%, lung disease in 37%, and pulmonary embolism in 1%. 55% of patients had more than one etiological diagnosis of AKI.The etiological diagnoses of AKI are represented in the following table (Table VI):

Table VI: Etiological diagnoses of acute respiratory failure

Etiological diagnoses of ARF	Workforce	%
DABPCO by superinfection bronchial	18	24
DABPCO by ICA	14	19
DABPCO by pneumopathy	10	13
DABPCO by ICA and pneumopathy	12	16
Isolated ICA	14	19
ICA by pneumopathy	5	7
Isolated lung disease	1	1
Pulmonary embolism	1	1

IRA:insufficiency respiratory failure acute respiratory failure; DABPCO: decompensation acute of chronic obstructive pulmonary disease; ACF: acute heart failure

The factors for decompensation of ICA are represented in the table below (Table VII):

Table VII: The factors of decompensation of acute heart failure

Factors in the decompensation of ICA	%
SCA	22
Hypertensive emergency	11
Bronchopulmonary infection	57
Rhythm disorder	11
Speed difference	2

ACI: acute heart failure; ACS: acute coronary syndrome.

III-Therapeutic management

III.1. The treatments administered

Drug treatments prescribed for etiological purposes were furosemide for 66% of patients, nebulized bricanyl and atrovent as well as hydrocortisone hemisuccinate for 73%, and antibiotic treatment for 69% of cases.Other treatments were dinitrate isosorbide for 11% and amiodarone for 10% of cases. 1% of patients required the use of vasoactive drugs.

III.2. Ventilatory treatment by non-invasive ventilation

Non-invasive ventilation was performed according to the VS-AI-PEP mode for 85% of cases and according to the CPAP mode for 15% for a mean duration of 7 hours (±6).

IV-Patient progress and referral

IV.1. Clinical course and referral of patients

Clinical success of NIV was observed in 68% of patients with 61% discharged home and 7% transferred to a pulmonary or cardiac ward after weaning from NIV for at least 24 hours. Among the 61% discharged at home, 5% required long-term oxygen therapy. In addition, 8% of the patients were hospitalized in intensive care and the use of intubation concerned 1.3% of patients. The in-hospital mortality rate was 24%. NIV failure thus concerned 32% of patients.

Table VIII: Patient progress and referral

Orientation/Evolution	%
Transfer to intensive care	8
Transfer to pneumology or cardiology	7
Going home	61
In-hospital mortality	24

IV.2. Length of stay

The duration of hospitalization in the emergency room was less than 24 hours for 20% of cases and more than 24 hours for 80%, with a median duration of 48 hours, a minimum duration of 5 hours and a maximum duration of 125 hours.

V- Prognostic factors

The correlation of clinical parameters to in-hospital mortality was studied. The clinical factors correlated with the risk of in-hospital mortality in univariate analysis were history of hypertension (p=0.026), hepato-jugular reflux (p=0.028) and IMO (p=0.016). The etiological diagnoses of AKI did not correlate with mortality risk (p>0.05). The biological prognostic factors that emerged in our study were blood urea>0.45g/L (p=0.005), CRP>10mg/L (p=0.004) and initial pH (p=0.044).

Table IX: Correlation of sociodemographic and background parameters to in-hospital mortality

Parameters	Group survivors	Deceased group	P
Type			0,246
male	43	11	
female	14	7	
Age groups			0,308
65-69	10	1	
70-79	33	10	
80-89	4	7	
Background			
COPD			0,251
yes	40	10	
no	17	8	
Heart failure			0,87
yes	17	5	
no	40	13	
Coronary insufficiency			1
yes	12	3	
no	45	15	
Atrial fibrillation			0,53
yes	17	4	
no	40	14	
Renal insufficiency			1
yes	15	5	
no	42	13	
HTA			0,026
yes	33	5	
no	24	13	

COPD: chronic obstructive pulmonary disease; hypertension: high blood pressure

Table X: Correlation ofparameters respiratoryinitial toin-hospital mortality

Parameters	Group survivors	Group deceased	p
SpO2<80			0,876
yes	21	7	
no	36	11	
SpO2 80-85%.			0,05
yes	9	7	
no	48	11	
SpO2 85-89%.			0,11
yes	21	3	
no	36	15	
SpO2>90			1
yes	6	1	
no	51	17	
FR<20 cycles/minute			0,57
yes	2	1	
no	55	17	
20-24 cycles/minute			0,086
yes	2	3	
no	55	15	
25-29 cycles/minute			0,892
yes	20	6	
no	37	12	
>30c/min			0,32
yes	33	8	
no	24	10	
Signs of struggle			1
yes	47	15	
no	10	3	

SpO2: peripheral oxygen saturation; RF: respiratory rate

Table XI : Correlation of cardiovascular cardiovascular parameters à in-hospital mortality			
Parameters	Survivor Group	Deceased group	p
RHJ			0,028
yes	6	6	
no	49	11	
TSJ			0,35
yes	16	7	
no	39	10	
IMO			0,016
yes	21	12	
no	35	5	
PAS>180mm Hg			0,28
yes	10	1	
no	47	17	
DBP>90mmHg			1
yes	7	2	
no	50	16	
Fc >120cpm			
yes	14	6	0,67
no	42	12	
Fc 90-120cpm			0,66
yes	32	12	
no	24	6	
Fc<90cpm			0,162
yes	9	0	
no	47	18	
no	55	15	
RHJ: hepato-jugular reflux; TSJ: spontaneous jugular junction; OMI: lower limb oedema; PAS: systolic blood pressure, DBP: blood pressure diastolic; Fc: heart rate			

Table XII: Correlation of neurological signs with in-hospital mortality			
Parameters	Survivor Group	Deceased group	p
SG ≤8			0,086
yes	2	3	
no	55	15	
SG 9-14			1
yes	13	4	
no	44	14	
SG to 15			0,31
yes	42	11	
no	15	7	
Temperature> 38°C			0,92
yes	12	3	
no	33	11	

SG: Glasgow score

Table XIII: Correlation of biological parameters with in-hospital mortality

Features	Group survivors	Deceased group	P
Urea>0.45g/L			0,005
yes	34	18	
no	21	0	
Creatinine>12mg/L			0,72
yes	28	9	
no	27	9	
Hemoglobinemia< 10g/dl			0,775
yes	6	3	
no	47	14	
WBC>10000/mm3			0,16
yes	34	15	
no	19	2	
WBC<4000/mm3			1
yes	4	1	
no	53	17	
CRP>10mg/L			0,004
yes	33	18	
no	17	0	

WBC: white blood cells; CRP: C-reactive protein

Initial pH was significantly correlated with mortality (p=0.044)

On the other hand, capnia was not significantly correlated with mortality (p=0.46).

Table XIV: Correlation of AKI etiologies with in-hospital mortality

Features	Group survivors	Group deceased	P
DABPCO superinfection			1
yes	14	4	
no	43	14	
DABPCO ICA			1
yes	11	3	
no	46	15	
DABPCO PNP			0,435
yes	9	1	
no	48	17	
Isolated ICA			1
yes	11	3	
no	46	15	
ICA PNP			0,588
yes	3	2	
no	54	16	
PNP			1
yes	1	0	
no	56	18	
EP			1
yes	1	0	
no	56	18	

DABPCO: acute decompensation of chronic obstructive pulmonary disease; ICA: acute heart failure; PNP: pneumonia; PE: pulmonary embolism.

DISCUSSION

The results of our study showed that out of seventy-five patients collected, aged over sixty-five years and requiring NIV, 55% of the patients had more than one etiological diagnosis of ARF.The etiological diagnoses selected were DABPCO in 72% of patients, CIA in 61%, pneumopathy in 37%, and pulmonary embolism in 1% of cases.Clinical success of non-invasive ventilatory treatment was observed in 68% of patients, 61% of whom were discharged home. The in-hospital mortality rate was 24% and 8% of patients were transferred to an intensive care unit. In addition, invasive ventilation was used in 1.3% of patients.Clinical factors correlated with mortality risk in univariate analysis were: history of hypertension (p=0.026), hepato-jugular reflux (p=0.028) and IMO (p=0.016). The biological factors were blood urea (p=0.005), CRP (p=0.004) and initial pH (p=0.044).Initial clinical signs of respiratory distress, etiological diagnosis of ARF, and Charlson index were not correlated with mortality risk (p>0.05).

I- General characteristics of the study population

- **Age**

The elderly population continues to grow each year, as part of the global phenomenon of aging (1.7).The National Institute on Aging (NIA) estimates that people over 65 years of age now represent 8% of the world's population (7). Because of their frailty and more frequent age-related pathologies, they are more often in need of care (2,8). Indeed, the number of elderly patients requiring hospitalization or intensive care is increasing significantly (9). However, these patients most often enter the hospital through the emergency department (1).According to the WHO, the elderly subject is defined by a chronological age greater than 65 years (2). In our study, we included patients meeting this criterion (1,2). A recent review of the literature concerning NIV in the elderly focused on this same age category, i.e. over 65 years (9).In fact, in the United States, the NIA defines three types of elderly: the This last group would represent 7% of the elderly population, and would include the "young old" or "young old" whose age is between 65 and 75 years, the "old old" or "old old" whose age is between 75 and 85 years, and the "very old" or "oldest old" who are older than 85 years (7,10). This last group would represent 7% of the elderly population. In the literature, studies carried out in elderly subjects with ARF using NIV have focused on different age groups (11-13). Among them, one study compared the three age groups defined by the NIA and included 56.2% of patients over 75 years of age (13). In our study, this group represented 50.7% of patients.

- **Pathological history**

According to a large systematic review of studies in seven high-income countries, more than half of all older people have multimorbidity, with a high prevalence in very old age (14).In our study, the median Charlson index was 5, which marks a terrain often heavy with comorbidities with as the most frequent antecedents, COPD disease (67%) and hypertension (51%). Our results showed a higher Charlson index than comparable studies in the literature (12).

- **Etiological diagnoses of acute respiratory failure**

ARF is a frequent complication in elderly subjects, particularly in those with chronic cardiopulmonary disease (15).A prospective observational study showed that the main diagnoses found among elderly patients presenting with AKI in the emergency department were CIA, pneumonia, DABPCO, pulmonary embolism and asthma (16).In our study, the etiologies of ARF were, in order of frequency, DABPCO (72%), ICA (61%), pneumonia (37%) and pulmonary embolism

(1%).In addition, there were no cases of asthma attacks with NIV during the study period.

II- Difficulties encountered in the management of elderly patients with ARF in the emergency department

- **Physiological and physiopathological particularities of the elderly subject**

Elderly subjects are complex, characterized by a great diversity of their health status and functional level. They are fragile, at risk of losing their autonomy at any time after an acute situation.

Their critical state often presents itself as a functional decompensation, a "confusion, depression, fall or nutritional decompensation" (1). This decompensation is caused by the onset of chronic and/or acute illnesses on a terrain more or less weakened by aging.

Several elements can add up to decompensation of a function (17):

o The effects of aging that progressively reduce functional reserves without in themselves causing decompensation.

o Additional chronic conditions that impair function.

o The factors of decompensation are often multiple and associated in the same patient: acute medical conditions, iatrogenic pathology and psychological stress.

During decompensation of respiratory function, the effects of aging are reflected in age-related physiological changes in lung function and the cardiovascular system (18).

▪ Diagnostic difficulties

The semiology of the elderly is often atypical and misleading, which may explain the difficulties of the diagnostic approach, particularly during dyspnea, the main symptom of ARF and a frequent reason for consultation of the elderly in the emergency room (18).Indeed, among the clinical presentations, cardiac asthma is more frequent in the elderly and, despite the presence of bronchospasm, reflects an acute decompensation of heart failure (18,19). Similarly, the diagnosis of pneumopathy is often difficult to establish, firstly clinically, because of the possible absence of fever, but also because of pre-existing radiological anomalies (18,20).On the other hand, diagnostic difficulties are linked to the often intertwined polypathology or "multimorbidities" of the elderly subject (1, 2, 8, 18).According to WHO, it is essential to consider not only the presence of specific diseases individually, but more importantly how they interact (2,21,22).In our study, several etiologies were often found in the same patient. Indeed, more than half of the patients (55%) had more than one etiological diagnosis for their AKI. The diagnoses ICA, DABPCO and pneumopathy were thus often associated.

▪ Therapeutic difficulties

When an elderly patient with ARF presents in the emergency department, it is essential to rapidly institute appropriate etiological treatment. When the patient presents with several etiologies, the clinician must ensure that the different therapies are tolerated.Also, the risk of drug interactions in older adults with comorbidities, may limit the use of potentially beneficial pharmacological treatments (23). Innovative approaches are therefore needed to identify the best treatments indicated for older adults with comorbidities (2).Etiological treatment with medication must be associated with ventilatory treatment. Among the techniques of respiratory assistance, NIV can be indicated in the elderly subject after eliminating the contraindications (5). The choice of mode and parameters differs according to the etiology, as do the therapeutic objectives.

Consequently, ventilatory treatment may also present certain difficulties related to the polypathology of the elderly subject.Thus, when practicing NIV, the CPAP mode, indicated during an ICA, may aggravate a DABPCO. Indeed, a high oxygen flow rate can aggravate hypoventilation in case of chronic hypoventilation. As for the level of PEEP, it can increase the risk of occurrence of barotrauma in this situation. The adaptation of the ventilatory parameters is thus done according to the therapeutic objectives related to the terrain, the causal pathology and finally the clinical response of the patient.

III-The use of NIV in the elderly in the emergency department: rationale for a therapeutic choice

The use of NIV is becoming increasingly widespread in the emergency department, particularly in the elderly (4). Indeed, this ventilatory technique makes it possible to prevent recourse to orotracheal intubation in many acute situations (9), and consequently reduces the risk of complications related to invasive ventilation, which are more likely to occur in the elderly (9,15,24,25).

On the other hand, NIV reduces the length of stay in hospital (26), which can be of great interest in emergency departments that often provide the entire management of elderly subjects suffering from ARF. This is due to the limited number of places in the resuscitation in public hospitals relative to the number of patients requiring intensive care.Furthermore, NIV can be indicated in many etiologies of ARF with an effectiveness that differs according to the diagnosis (26). Its efficacy has been widely established during CIA and DABPCO (5,15,26,27), often encountered in the elderly (16).

According to the recommendations of the European Respiratory Society and the American Thoracic Society published in 2017 concerning the clinical application of NIV during ARF, it is strongly indicated during DABPCO with hypercapnia. Indeed, it allows an improvement of the symptoms with correction of the respiratory acidosis. It also reduces the need for invasive ventilation, hospital stay and mortality (26). It is therefore a preferential choice for patients with acute respiratory acidosis, with close monitoring of patients and the possibility of rapid recourse to invasive ventilation in the event of non-improvement (26,28). In our study, DABPCO was very frequent, i.e. in 72% of patients.Concerning ICA, present in 61% of our patients, the data in the literature show that NIV allows to reduce the use of invasive ventilation during ICA and hospital mortality with similar effects for CPAP and VS-AI-PEP mode according to several studies (29,30,31,32).Finally, NIV is also indicated in other ARF situations, notably in immunocompromised patients, during care palliative, post-operative or post-traumatic context. We note that no recommendation has been issued concerning de novo ARF, severe acute asthma, and pandemic viral infection, based on data from the literature (26).

However, with regard to de novo ARF, some studies have identified populations likely to benefit from NIV with hypoxemic ARF, acute community-acquired lung disease and/or early acute respiratory distress syndrome, subject to pre-established conditions. Indeed, these patients must be managed by an experienced care team with close monitoring and early reassessment after initiation of NIV in order to decide on a rapid recourse to invasive ventilation in the absence of improvement. Finally, these patients must be well selected by excluding in particular those with consciousness disorders, organ dysfunctions and/or signs of shock (26). In our study, the diagnosis of lung disease was present in 37% of patients and was most often associated with DABPCO in 29% of cases and ICA in 7% of cases.

IV-Factors involved in reducing invasive ventilation in the elderly

In elderly subjects, ventilatory treatment of ARF is clearly associated with a decrease in the use of invasive ventilation (33,34).This phenomenon is multifactorial in origin, due in particular to better management of the ICA and DABPCO but also to decisions limitation of therapeutic care more widely taken in this age group (15,33).Indeed, since the goal of intensive care is to reduce morbidity and mortality by treating organ failure in the resuscitation setting, it is essential to take into consideration the patient's wishes regarding "end of life", the impact of comorbidities, loss of autonomy, and the prognosis of the disease (5,35,36). The presence of a poor prognosis, coupled with the deleterious risk of invasive ventilation and intensive care hospitalization, are all factors that are often involved in the decision to limit therapeutic care (33).In fact, the impact of intensity of care on survival in elderly subjects is still a matter of debate (24,37). Furthermore, it is certain that the decision not to intubate "DNI" cannot be considered an indication for NIV (9). However, the use of NIV for palliative purposes is becoming increasingly common (37,38).In our study, intubation was performed in only 1.3% of patients, while the in-hospital mortality rate was 24%. These results are consistent with this trend. Thus, advanced patient age and multiple comorbidities often influence the decision to limit therapeutic escalation. Furthermore, more than half of our patients were "old old" patients, i.e., patients who were "The average age of the patients was 74 years (min=65, max=88).Despite technological advances, the mortality rate increases with age, especially in the "oldest old" (35). According to one study, "very old patients", i.e. those over 85 years of age, are potentially "good candidates for a less invasive management strategy" (37).In addition, our population had a mean Charlson index of 5.15 (±1.6), which indicates a terrain often fraught with comorbidities, with COPD (67%) and hypertension (51%) as the most frequent antecedents. Other pathologies were also frequent, such as diabetes in nearly a third of the patients, heart failure in 29%, ACFA in 28% and renal failure in

27% of cases. The prevalence of multimorbidity increases with age and is associated with a higher mortality rate (39,40).

V- Clinical effectiveness of NIV in the elderly

Because of its clinical efficacy and good tolerance allowed by a non-invasive approach, NIV has become an essential technique in the management of ARF (41).However, in the literature, there are few data on its clinical effectiveness in the elderly (9,42). Indeed, there are not enough prospective randomized studies to justify the choice of the best treatment for ARF in the elderly (42).In any case, there seems to be no correlation between the clinical results of NIV practice and the age factor in view of the data (41). Indeed, studies have shown that the clinical efficacy of NIV during ARF was not dependent on age (11,12,37,43). An Italian prospective study comparing patients under 75 years of age and those over 75 years of age concluded that there was no significant difference in mortality rate and use of orotracheal intubation during hypercapnic ARF in COPD (11). Another Spanish study including patients over 75 years of age put on NIV for respiratory acidosis with pH<7.35 and capnia>45mmHg also showed no significant difference when comparing mortality rate with a group under 75 years (12). Our study showed clinical success of NIV evident in 68% of our patients of whom 61% were discharged home. In the literature, the results differ according to the inclusion criteria and show an overall failure rate of NIV in ARF of any cause ranging from 20 to 30% (44), with NIV failure being defined by the use of invasive ventilation or the occurrence of death (44). Furthermore, the results of our study are comparable to those of other studies (12,44). The in-hospital mortality rate was 24% with recourse to invasive ventilation in 1.3% of patients. This can be explained by the frequency of comorbidities in our series, a factor that could intervene in the decision to limit care.

Table XV: Comparison of clinical effectiveness of NIV in other studies

Authors	Type of study and year	Place of study	Membership and Patients		Judging criteria	Results %
Segrelles	Prospective	RMU	106	85>75 years	Mortality	21,4
Calvo,	2012					
(12)				21<75	Mortality	21,7
Çiftci, (13)	Prospective	Resuscitation	162	>65 years old	Mortality	18
	2017				IOT	24,6
Nicolini,	Prospective	Emergency RMU	207	121>75 years	Mortality	19,8
(11)	2014				IOT	10,7
				86<75 years	Mortality	10,4
					IOT	11,6
Our	Retrospective	emergencies	75	> 65 years old	Mortality	24
study,	2017				IOT	1,3

RMU: respiratory monitoring unit; IOT: orotracheal intubation

VI- Prognostic factors

In the literature, the success of NIV is inversely related to the number and severity of comorbidities, the state of consciousness and the early resolution of signs of respiratory distress (9).In our study, the clinical factors correlated with the risk of mortality in univariate analysis were: history of hypertension (p=0.026), hepato-jugular reflux (p=0.028) and IMO (p=0.016).Indeed, signs of right heart failure may reflect the severity of COPD disease, indicating a pulmonary heart stage chronic and thus a sign of severity related to the terrain (45). During CIA, the presence of hepato-jugular reflux correlates with an occlusive pulmonary artery pressure greater than 20 mmHg (18,46,47).

Concerning the etiological diagnosis of ARF, our results did not show a significant correlation with the risk of mortality, the same was true for the Charlson index.Finally, several biological prognostic factors emerged from this study in univariate analysis. This is the case for blood urea (p=0.005), CRP (p=0.004) and initial pH (p=0.044).In another recent study in patients over 65 years of age with hypercapnic ARF, initial pH and CRP were also prognostic factors in the DABPCO and ICA groups. Among other factors, GCS score, APACHE II score and severity of dyspnea were independent predictors of NIV failure (13).

VII- Limitations of the study and perspectives

Our study was retrospective, which may have had several limitations.The delay in the initiation of NIV, considered as a prognostic factor, was variable, depending on the clinical evolution of the patients, but also sometimes on the logistic conditions.On the other hand, it would have been interesting to compare the clinical results observed in the elderly versus patients under 65 years of age and to perform a subgroup analysis in order to better evaluate the effectiveness of NIV in the elderly and to identify patients who may benefit more from it in the emergency department.Moreover, the practice of NIV can sometimes be difficult, due to the lack of equipment but also of medical and paramedical staff, hence the importance of reinforcing all the necessary means to optimize the management of elderly patients with ARF in the emergency room.Finally, the clinical effectiveness of NIV is conditioned by the level of experience of the medical and paramedical team (41). It is therefore essential to encourage continuing education of health professionals in the field of respiratory assistance by devoting a specific section to the management of the elderly population.

The management of elderly patients presenting with ARF in the emergency department can be exposed to various difficulties. This is due to the frailty of these patients due to ageing, but also to the multiple comorbidities whose prevalence increases with age.The difficulties are of a diagnostic nature, linked to the atypical symptomatology and the polypathology of the elderly subject, but they are also of a therapeutic nature. Indeed, the therapeutic strategy differs according to the causal pathology. In the elderly, it is therefore essential to understand how the different etiologies of ARF interact in the same patient in order to adapt the treatment and prevent potential complications.The treatment is both etiological and symptomatic, requiring respiratory assistance for the patient whose prognosis is imminently committed. In this context, the use of NIV, which is becoming more and more widespread in emergencies, can be a good alternative for respiratory assistance. Its effectiveness has been widely established during CIA and DABPCO, etiological diagnoses particularly frequent in the elderly subject.The objectives of this work were to study the characteristics of non-invasive ventilatory treatment in the elderly subject admitted to the emergency department for ARF and to highlight the predictive factors.We conducted a retrospective study including seventy-five patients aged over sixty-five years with a median age of 74 years with a minimum age of 65 years and a maximum age of 88 years. Our results showed a male predominance with a sex ratio of 2.57. The median Charlson index was 5 with a minimum of 3 and a maximum of 9. The etiological diagnoses retained were DABPCO in 72% of the cases, ICA in 61%, pneumopathy in 37% and pulmonary embolism in 1% of cases.Successful NIV was observed in 68% of our patients, 61% of whom were discharged home. Failure of NIV resulted in an in-hospital mortality rate of 24% and hospitalization in the intensive care unit in 8% of patients. Invasive ventilation was used in only 1.3% of patients. Thus, the frequency of comorbidities was a factor that could have influenced the decision to limit care.

Despite this, our mortality rate was comparable to other studies (12,44). The clinical factors correlated with the risk of mortality in univariate analysis were history of hypertension, hepato-jugular reflux and IMO (p<0.05). Regarding the initial clinical signs of respiratory distress and the etiological diagnosis of ARF, our results did not show a significant correlation to the risk of mortality. The same was true for the Charlson index.However, the frequent association of acute comorbidities highlighted in our series could explain, on a pathophysiological basis, the difficulties encountered during the practice of NIV.In addition, several biological prognostic factors emerged from this study such as blood urea, CRP and initial pH (p<0.05). These last two factors have also been identified in the literature (13).Thus, our study showed that many difficulties can be associated with the non-invasive ventilatory treatment of elderly patients with ARF in the emergency department. However, this treatment remains interesting, allowing to avoid as much as possible the complications of invasive ventilation, a technique sometimes considered too aggressive for patients with heavy comorbidities. Finally, as the therapeutic management of elderly subjects with ARF takes place essentially in the emergency room, it is more than necessary to improve the logistical conditions of these services in order to optimize the use of this technique and improve the prognosis of these patients.

REFERENCES

1- Duquesne F. Vulnerability of the elderly. Urgences. 2011;(28):277-91.

2- Beard J, Officer A, Cassels A, Bustreo F, Worning AM, Asamoa-Baah A, et al. World report on aging and health. Geneva: World Health Organization; 2016. pp. 1-296.

3 Perrin C, Jullien V, Lemoigne F. Practical and technical aspects of noninvasive ventilation. Rev Mal Respir. 2004;21(3):556-66.

4- Combes X, Jabre P, Vivien B, Carli P. Non-invasive ventilation in emergency medicine. Annales Françaises De Médecine d'Urgence. 2011;1:260-6.

5- French Society of Anesthesia and Intensive Care, French Language Pneumology Society, French Language Intensive Care Society. Non-invasive ventilation in acute respiratory failure (excluding neonates). 3ème Conférence de Consensus. Paris: SFAR, SPLF, SRLF; 2006.

6- Roch A, Mercier E. An update on invasive mechanical ventilation - Main ventilatory modes in invasive mechanical ventilation in adults. Resuscitation. 2011;20 Suppl2:S530-S4.

7- Li RM, Ladarola AC, Maisano CC. Why population aging matters: a global perspective. U.S. Department of Health and Human Services; 2007. p. 1-32.

8- Henrard JC. Health in old age. Public Health News and Issues. 1997;(20):2-11.

9- Piroddi IMG, Barlascini C, Esquinas A, Braido F, Banfi P, Nicolini A. Non-invasive mechanical ventilation in elderly patients: A narrative review. Geriatr Gerontol Int. 2017;17(5):689-96.

10- Lalive d'Epinay C, Spini D. Old age: a recent field of research. Gerontology and Society. 2007;123:31-54.

11- Nicolini A, Santo M, Ferrera L, Ferrari-Bravo M, Barlascini C, Perazzo A. The use of non-invasive ventilation in very old patients with hypercapnic acute respiratory failure because of COPD exacerbation. Int J Clin Pract.

2014;68(12):1523-9.

12- Segrelles Calvo G, Zamora García E, Girón Moreno R, Vázquez Espinosa E, Gómez Punter RM, Fernandes Vasconcelos G, et al. Non-invasive ventilation in an elderly population admitted to a respiratory monitoring unit: causes, complications and one-year evolution. Arch Bronconeumol. 2012;48(10):349-54.

13- Çiftci F, Çiledağ A, Erol S. Non-invasive ventilation for acute hypercapnic respiratory failure in older patients. Wien Klin Wochenschr. 2017;129(19-20):680-6.

14- Marengoni A, Angleman S, Melis R, Mangialasche F, Karp A, Garmen A, et al. Aging with multimorbidity: a systematic review of the literature. Ageing Res Rev. 2011;10(4):430-9.

15- Scala R. Challenges on non-invasive ventilation to treat acute respiratory failure in the elderly. BMC Pulm Med. 2016;16(1):150.

16- Ray P, Birolleau S, Lefort Y, Becquemin MH, Beigelman C, Isnard R, et al. Acute respiratory failure in the elderly: etiology, emergency diagnosis and prognosis. Crit Care. 2006;10(3):R82.

17- Bouchon J.P. 1 + 2 + 3 or how to try to be efficient in geriatrics? Rev Prat. 1984;34:888-92.

18- Ray P, Birolleau S, Riou B. Acute dyspnea in the elderly. Rev Mal Respir. 2004;21(5):842.

19- Snashall PD, Chung KF. Airway obstruction and bronchial hyperresponsiveness in left ventricular failure and mitral stenosis. Am Rev Respir Dis. 1991;144(4):945- 56.

20- Prendki V, Huttner B, Perrier A, Reny JL, Stirnemann J. Pneumonia in the elderly: are there any specificities? Rev Med Suisse. 2014;10(449):2081-6.

21- Ham C. The ten characteristics of the high-performing chronic care system. Health Econ Policy Law. 2010;5(Pt 1):71-90.

22- Eklund K, Wilhelmson K. Outcomes of coordinated and integrated interventions targeting frail elderly people: a systematic review of randomised controlled trials. Health Soc Care Community. 2009; 17(5):447-58.

23- DuBeau CE, Kuchel GA, Johnson T, Palmer MH, Wagg A. Incontinence in the frail elderly: report from the 4th International Consultation on Incontinence. Neurourol Urodyn. 2010;29(1):165-78.

24- Esteban A, Anzueto A, Frutos-Vivar F, Alía I, Ely EW, Brochard L, et al. Outcome of older patients receiving mechanical ventilation. Intensive Care Med. 2004;30(4):639-46.

25- Pingleton SK. Complications of acute respiratory failure. Am Rev Respir Dis. 1988;137(6):1463-93.

26- Rochwerg B, Brochard L, Elliott MW, Hess D, Hill NS, Nava S, et al. Official ERS/ATS clinical practice guidelines: noninvasive ventilation for acute respiratory failure. Eur Respir J. 2017;50(2)1602426.

27- Mosier JM, Hypes C, Joshi R, Whitmore S, Parthasarathy S, Cairns CB. Ventilator Strategies and Rescue Therapies for Management of Acute Respiratory Failure in the Emergency Department. Ann Emerg Med. 2015;66(5):529-41.

28- Scarpazza P, Incorvaia C, Melacini C, Cattaneo R, Bonacina C, Riario-Sforza GG, et al. Shrinking the room for invasive ventilation in hypercapnic respiratory failure. Int J COPD. 2013;8:135-7.

29- Cabrini L, Landoni G, Oriani A, Plumari VP, Nobile L, Greco M, et al. Noninvasive ventilation and survival in acute care settings: a comprehensive systematic review and metaanalysis of randomized controlled trials. Crit Care Med. 2015;43(4):880-8.

30- Gray A, Goodacre S, Newby DE, Masson M, Sampson F, Nicholl J, et al. Noninvasive ventilation in acute cardiogenic pulmonary edema. N Engl J Med. 2008;359(2):142-51.

31- Potts JM. Noninvasive positive pressure ventilation: effect on mortality in acute cardiogenic pulmonary edema: a pragmatic meta-analysis. Pol Arch Med Wewn. 2009;119(6):349-53.

32- Plaisance P, Pirracchio R, Berton C, Vicaut E, Payen D. A randomised study of out-hospital continuous positive airway pressure for acute cardiogenic pulmonary oedema: physiological and clinical effects. Eur Heart J. 2007;28(23):2823-4.

33- Vargas N, Esquinas AM. The reduced use of intubations in elderly patients in the emergency department: Many insights behind a historical trend. Am J Emerg Med. 2018;36(12)2321.

34- Johnson T, Richman P, Allegra JR, Eskin B, Seger J. Intubations in elderly patients have decreased from 1999 through 2014-Results of a multi-center cohort study. Am J Emerg Med. 2018;36(11):1964-6.

35- Vargas N, Tibullo L, Landi E, Carifi G, Pirone A, Pippo A, et al. Caring for critically ill older patients: a clinical review. Aging Clin Exp Res. 2017;29(5):833- 45.

36- Garrouste-Orgeas M, Timsit JF, Montuclard L, Colvez A, Gattolliat O, Philippart F, et al. Decision-making process, outcome, and 1-year quality of life of octogenarians referred for intensive care unit admission. Intensive Care Med. 2006;32(7):1045-51.

37- Schortgen F, Follin A, Piccari L, Roche-Campo F, Carteaux G, Taillandier-Heriche E, et al. Results of non-invasive ventilation in very old patients. Ann Intensive Care. 2012;2(1):5.

38- Perrin C, Jullien V, Duval Y, Defrance C. Place of noninvasive ventilation in palliative and end-of-life care. Rev Mal Respir. 2008;25(10):1227-36.

39- Van den Akker M, Buntinx F, Metsemakersl JFM, Roos S, Knottnerus JA. Multimorbidity in general practice: prevalence, incidence, and determinants of co-occurring chronic and recurrent diseases. J Clin Epidemiol. 1998;51(5):367-75.

40- Gijsen R, Hoeymans N, Schellevis FG, Ruwaard D, Satariano WA, Van den Bos GA. Causes and consequences of comorbidity: a review. J Clin Epidemiol. 2001;54(7):661-74.

41- Cuvelier A, Benhamou D, Muir JF. Noninvasive ventilation of elderly patients in the intensive care unit. Rev Mal Respir. 2003;20(3):399-410.

42- Nava S, Grassi M, Fanfulla F, Domenighetti G, Carlucci A, Perren A, et al. Non- invasive ventilation in elderly patients with acute hypercapnic respiratory failure: a randomised controlled trial. Ageing. 2011;40(4): 444-50.

43- Ozsancak Ugurlu A, Sidhom SS, Khodabandeh A, Ieong M, Mohr C, Lin DY, et al. Use and Outcomes of Noninvasive Ventilation for Acute Respiratory Failure in Different Age Groups. Respir Care. 2016;61(1):36-43.

44- Lari F, Pilati G, Bragagni G, Di Battista N. Use of non-invasive ventilation for acute respiratory failure in general medical wards. Eur J of Intern Med. 2008;19(1):s10-s11.

45- Chaouat A. Chronic pulmonary heart in COPD. Rev Mal Respir. 2009;26(10):1184-5.

46- Stevenson LW, Perloff JK. The limited availability of physical signs for estimating hemodynamics in chronic heart failure. JAMA. 1989;261(6):884-8.

47- Butman SM, Emy GA, Standen JR, Kern KB, Hahn E. Bedside cardiovascular examination in patients with severe chronic heart failure: importance of rest or inducible jugular venous distension. J Am Coll Cardiol. 1993;22(4):968-74.

APPENDIXES

THE CHARLSON COMORBIDITY INDEX

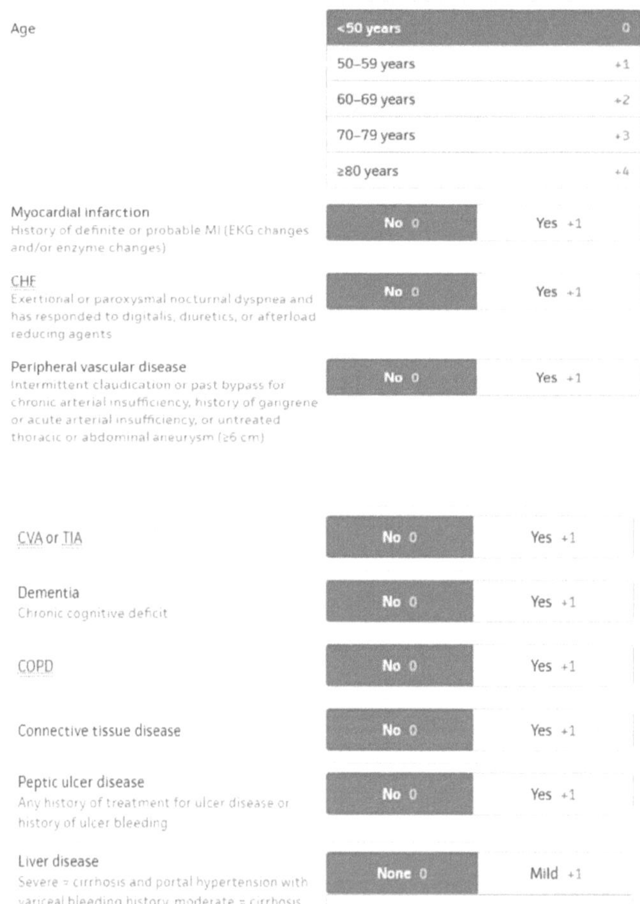

Diabetes mellitus	**None or diet-controlled**	0
	Uncomplicated	+1
	End-organ damage	+2

| Hemiplegia | **No** 0 | Yes +2 |

Moderate to severe CKD
Severe = on dialysis, status post kidney
transplant, uremia, moderate = creatinine >3
mg/dL (0.27 mmol/L)

| Moderate to severe CKD | **No** 0 | Yes +2 |

| Solid tumor | **None** 0 | Localized +2 | Metastatic +6 |

| Leukemia | **No** 0 | Yes +2 |

| Lymphoma | **No** 0 | Yes +2 |

| AIDS | **No** 0 | Yes +6 |

Total	Probabilité de survie à 10 ans
0	99%
1	96%
2	90%
3	77%
4	53%
5	21%
6	2%
>6	0%